Yoga

Easy Beginners Yoga Poses Guide, Reduce Anxiety, Stress, Sharpen Your Mind, Learn Yoga, Benefits of Yoga

Yoga

This document is geared towards providing exact and reliable information in regards to the topic and issue covered. The publication is sold with the idea that the publisher is not required to render accounting, officially permitted, or otherwise, qualified services. If advice is necessary, legal or professional, a practiced individual in the profession should be ordered.

- From a Declaration of Principles which was accepted and approved equally by a Committee of the American Bar Association and a Committee of Publishers and Associations.

The information herein is offered for informational purposes solely, and is universal as so. The presentation of the information is without contract or any type of guarantee assurance.

Introduction

I want to thank you and congratulate you for downloading the book, *"Yoga: Easy Beginners Yoga Poses Guide, Reduce Anxiety, Stress, Sharpen Your Mind, Learn Yoga, Benefits of Yoga"*.

This book has actionable yoga poses for complete beginners to help you combat stress and anxiety as well as sharpen your mind.

In the past few years, yoga has been increasing in popularity tremendously. In fact, it has become so popular that there are plans to include yoga as an Olympics sport! The question that you may probably ask yourself is; why should someone spend their time and energy learning how to perform some of the crazy stunts that yoga is often associated with? Does it have any benefit to the average Joe? If there are any benefits, do you have to do the impossible stunts just to derive the benefits that come from yoga? Is there any scientific proof that supports why you should practice yoga?

Well, this book will answer this and many other questions. In particular, you will learn how to use yoga to combat stress and anxiety as well as master how to use it to sharpen your mind.

Thanks again for downloading this book, I hope you enjoy it!

Table of Contents

Yoga: An Introduction

Yoga is an ancient system of practices, principles and philosophies that are derived from the Vedic tradition of the Himalayas and India dating back as early as 2500 years ago. The system recognizes the multi-dimensional nature of the human person and usually primarily relates to the very nature and workings of the human mind based on self-enquiry and experiential practice.

The word yoga is derived from a Sanskrit root word 'yuj', which essentially means 'to yoke'- as in oxen, or 'to join' the spirit and the body together. In other words, you can think of it as joining the body, the mind and the spirit.

In contemporary terms, you can think of yoga as 'union'. But then you may ask; union of what?

The truth is; there is no one particular definition of this union; it all depends on your perspective whether spiritual, religious, scientific or practical. Let's take a quick look at some common unions that people usually seek:

✓ The union of 'yin' and 'yang'

✓ The union of 'higher self' and 'lower self'

✓ The union of the spirit, mind and body

✓ The union of your 'true nature' and your 'everyday nature'

✓ The union of female and male side

- ✓ The union of the divine and the individual soul

- ✓ The union of your unconscious and the conscious mind or bringing your unconscious mind into full awareness

Therefore, yoga essentially is all about 'union'. According to a sage who was named Patanjali:

1. You can think of yoga as the control of the vrittis of your mind

Vrittis in this case are the modifications or waves within your mind. For instance, you can think of such 'waves' like emotions, memories, thoughts etc. Although these waves are not evil or bad, but like the waves of a lake usually scatter the light and make it hard to see your reflection, the vrittis of your mind make it hard for you to see your true self. In addition:

2. When you control these vrittis, the seer usually abides in his true nature

You can think of it this way; every single thing in the universe has its 'true nature' i.e. the essence that usually comes forth whenever you let things to be in their own natural environment. For instance:

- ✓ A mountain is usually still in its natural environment while

- ✓ Water is cool

- ✓ Fire is usually consuming

✓ Diamond is usually hard

✓ A piece of coal is usually black

So, what exactly is our true nature as humans? What's your true nature? If you are searching for this i.e. trying to be one with your true nature, you are a yogi (male) or a yogini (female). Basically, yoginis and sages from different parts of the world and with different practices agree that the true nature of human being is peace, bliss and happiness. They agree that our true nature of humans is that we are truly divine.

Having been in existence for thousands of years, it (yoga) has evolved to take different disciplines and styles. In fact, just because someone is yogi or is studying yoga doesn't mean that you know anything about them. The truth is that there are very many ways through which someone can practice yoga. You can think of it this way; when someone tells you they are a scientist, you don't just assume that they spend all time at the lab or outdoors gazing at the stars or studying animals? Just as there are many branches of science that someone can pursue, the same applies to yoga; some can spend all day dancing and singing to Hare Krishna, some can spend time meditating, some can spend time praying, some contemplating and some doing other things; there is just no one way of practicing yoga!

What does it entail?

In yoga, the mind, the breath and the body are usually seen as multi-dimensional aspects of every human being. It is through the different yoga techniques that you cultivate your experience of that union resulting to a far greater integration of internal peacefulness, being and clarity of your mind. You can think of it as a system, which is designed to cultivate happiness, health and a far greater sense of higher consciousness and self awareness. Through yoga, you can cultivate health, & wellbeing (social, mental, emotional and physical) through practicing different techniques that include breathing exercises, breathe awareness, relaxation and concentration, meditation and self-inquiry, and postures and movement.

Yoga is more than mere exercise and fitness regime. It is a way towards positive living that enriches the body, the mind and the soul in totality. Yoga fine tunes the body's balance, mental state and spiritual character.

Yoga is an amalgamation of four aspects namely –

1. Asanas/poses

2. Pranayamas

3. Meditation

4. Diet

Let's explain these 4 in detail:

Yoga Poses/Asanas

Asana simply means pose or posture. It literally means 'seat'. When yoga started, there was only one asana, which was essentially a stable as well as comfortable pose meant for prolonged seated meditation. Yoga is known to open the energy channels (nadis) as well as psychic centers (chakras) of your body besides just toning and stretching your physical body. Additionally, different yoga poses usually purify as well as calm, control and focus your mind. This is so because various categories of postures usually produce various physical, emotional, mental as well as energetic effects. Here are some of the effects:

✓ Yoga poses are a way to exercise your body's internal as well as external organs.

✓ Different yoga postures improve blood circulation and trigger 'happiness hormones' for rejuvenation.

✓ By performing yoga poses, body organs get stretched, strengthened and stimulated, which leads to unblocking of body's seven chakras. Chakras are the seven focal points in human body through which energy flows. These 7 chakras are –

1. Root Chakra – This is located on the base area of spine's tailbone area and represents the foundation of our mind and intellect.

2. Sacral Chakra – This chakra is situated in the body's lower abdominal area and is associated with our sexuality, wellness and sense of abundant bounties in life.

3. Solar Plexus Chakra – This chakra is locate in body's upper abdominal area and regulates our confidence level.

4. Heart Chakra – It is situated right in the central portion of our chest and controls our ability to love.

5. Throat Chakra – It is located inside our throats and controls our communication skills.

6. Third Eye Chakra – This is situated right in between our two eyes and helps us focus well. It also makes us see life with a broad perspective.

7. Crown Chakra – This is considered to be the premium chakra that makes our conscious and spirits attain higher level. It is located in the crown of our head.

Chakras, as discussed above, are focal points of energy inside our bodies. Whenever, any of the chakras is blocked, the energy flow gets hampered and the life force gets stuck. Yoga can be effectively used for unblocking of our chakras so that fresh energy can flow in our veins, arteries and through our nerves. Kundalini Yoga is a great yoga technique that helps in awakening of energy force. In this case, while performing different yoga poses, you end up stretching different body parts as well as boost your chakras.

You can learn more about chakras here, here and here.

Pranayama

Pranayama refers to an ancient practice, which is usually concerned with breath control. It, pranayama, can also be referred to as the 'better half' of yoga discipline. It is a technique, which entails breathing in the right way; correct breathing techniques make a huge difference to our state of mind. In fact, practicing yoga without following the correct Pranayama techniques will not render the best results. Why is that so? Well, our body absorbs more oxygen and thus gets detoxified when you breathe properly. Consequently, a body free of toxins stays healthy and refreshed and consequently leads to positive thoughts. The basic tenets of Pranayama are –

- ✓ The best time for performing pranayama is early in the morning because of the fresh air that contains maximum oxygen

- ✓ Ensure you are on an empty stomach and with clean bowel system when practicing pranayama.

- ✓ Choose a quiet, well ventilated, uncluttered and clean room or a green area like the lawn or a garden

- ✓ Wear comfortable and loosely fitted clothes.

- ✓ Sit on a mat on the floor in squat posture. If sitting on floor is not possible, you can also sit on a chair

- ✓ Since Pranayama is associated with holding and releasing of breath, you should be careful when practicing yoga when suffering from asthma, congestion or hypertension. However, pranayama has been proven to relieve the symptoms of asthma, depression and anxiety.

- ✓ Strictly avoid smoking before or after pranayama

- ✓ Breathe normally through the nose without any jerks.

- ✓ Expand out your chest muscles during inhalation and inward at the time of exhalation

- ✓ Follow the basic pranayama pattern of - A long and deep inhalation - short pause with breath held up - a long and a deep exhalation. Ideally, this pattern should be in proportions of 1:4:2. This implies that you should be exhaling slowly than inhaling. You can learn more about how to practice pranayam here.

Note: Different yoga experts agree that you should practice pranayama when practicing different yoga poses. This is because while only pranayama can refresh the mind and body, it must be coupled with yoga poses if you are to derive many more benefits.

Meditation

Although the first thought about yoga is perhaps associated with physical manifestation of exercising, one inherent and comprehensive experience associated with yoga is of meditation, which usually generates awareness of self-existence. Meditation is a powerful doctrine of yoga that creates self-awareness of high order and usher in positive thinking into minds. In fact, regular meditation sessions during yoga practice awaken soulful perception and leave no room for negative thoughts.

Those who consider meditation to be a complicated practice often fail to meditate in the correct way or have wrong goals in their minds. Meditation isn't about finding something deep inside your mind and then stirring it. It is about learning to silence the non-stop chattering of our minds and evoking mindfulness.

At the time of meditating, close your eyes gently and focus on your breath. Gradually, the monkey mind will start settling down and your thinking process will get purified.

Right Diet

Yoga associates great importance to diet. Yoga practitioners believe that what we eat leaves a great impact on not just our bodies but also over our mind and soul. Yoga asserts; "We are what we eat". Here is what yoga practitioners agree about diet:

- ✓ Not to become slaves of taste and gluttony

- ✓ Strictly say no to fast food items for they cause obesity due to presence of excessive oils, sugar, artificial preservatives

- ✓ Select natural nutrients in foods like whole grains, vegetables, seasonal fruits, honey, milk, dry fruits etc

- ✓ Take seasonal fruits and /or its juice for they supply fiber to the body

- ✓ Eat 50 percent of your hunger; fill the remaining 25 percent with water and keep the rest of your stomach space empty

- ✓ Eat only when hungry and avoid snacks in between the meals

- ✓ Avoid spices, tea, coffee, salty food and alcoholic drinks for they weaken your mind and body

- ✓ Drink 10 - 12 glasses of water daily

These 4 guiding principles are great gateways to positive living. For this book, we will focus on yoga asanas for attaining different goals. As we've already stated, just because you are practicing the asanas doesn't mean that you don't implement the 3 other principles. Before we discuss how to use yoga for attaining different goals, let's first highlight the different benefits that you stand to derive through practicing yoga.

Why Yoga?

Even if you are new to yoga, you must be aware that yoga is not about jumping or doing vigorous kinds of exercises. Instead, yoga is an amalgamation of subtle exercising coupled with breathing techniques that relaxes muscles and tones up the body. In fact, yoga is the only workout option that gently massages internal organs and is just as good as any other physical activity like cardio. To help you understand this better as well as give you the motivation to do something, let's discuss some reasons why you should try yoga:

1. Yoga is enough workout

Yoga is a remarkable way to work out. To add on, it can be customized on the basis of age, gender, time and comfort level. Yoga poses are designed for working out the whole body (including the internal organs). In addition, they include effortless sequence of movements that become part of daily health care.

2. Yoga will help you to achieve a balanced and a positive outlook towards life and lifestyle

Yoga is beyond the general perception of being just a simple exercising discipline. In line with the literal meaning of 'union' yoga, conjoins humanity with divinity. Once yoga makes the body flexible, lean and lithe, it starts working on the mind and the soul with the help of pranayama and meditation.

3. Yoga can help you to control your breathing pattern

Yoga can help you in controlling your breathing pattern, which, as I already stated is an effective way to manage stress. Deep and mindful breathing feeds your body with good amount of oxygen that benefits body organs and our brain's neurons. Proper breathing, as I already stated, is a good remedy for such respiratory diseases like asthma.

4. For better sleep and relaxation

Yoga can help boost your body's relaxation, which can in turn help improve your sleep. So how does it do that? Well, yoga helps in sobering the mind and in easing joint or muscular pains that consequently helps in boosting your sleep. For you to attain that, you should try implementing the poses that help boost your calmness. We will highlight some of these asanas later in the book.

5. For developing physical as well as mental fortitude

Besides physical strength, yoga can build your mental fortitude amazingly. Once your body becomes flexible, and is able to exercise and you can meditate smoothly, you are likely to start noticing an improvement in overall vitality and vigor. While pranayama strengthens the lungs, yoga poses develop core strength with the help of stretches and lunges.

6. For becoming better and better

Yoga and meditation make a powerful combination that makes for a better life and living. Yoga poses bring in disciplined approach towards life and alter things for better while meditation improves our mental state by bringing peacefulness to the way we perceive the world.

7. Stress relief

Yoga entails several relaxation techniques that, if practiced regularly can help you a lot calmer. In addition, yoga can help you to start seeing the bigger picture and even act from integrity as opposed to freaking out.

8. Yoga can help boost your flexibility

You really don't need to do the crazy stunts to be considered a yoga enthusiast. Nonetheless, the physical postures often have different spinal twists that will loosen the many joints in your spine. This can ultimately improve your tennis game as well as your golf swing. In addition, you can be sure of improved detoxification and better digestion. You can think of your body as a sponge that has dirty sink water; if you twist gently, you end up wringing the sponge out and ultimately purging toxins.

Note: Obviously, the above list of benefits is in no way conclusive. The list of benefits that yoga can bring to you is endless. Here is a more comprehensive list of these benefits:

Physical Benefits

- Lessens chronic pains

- Yoga helps control abnormal blood pressure

Yoga

- Yoga can help cure insomnia

- Yoga enhances flexibility

- Strong bones, joints and toned muscles

- Yoga helps to clear your respiratory tract

- Yoga can help improve your energy and vitality

- Yoga can balance your metabolism

- Weight management

- Better Cardio health

- Improved agility and physical performance

- Prevention of internal injury

- Lowers cholesterol

- Regulates blood glucose levels

- Improves lipid profile

- Diminishes asthma

- Treats Thyroid disorders

- Increase in count of red blood cells

- Prevents osteoporosis

- Supplies more oxygen to cells

- Aids quick recovery from diseases

- Detoxifies the body

- Results to better hair growth

- Develops motor skills

- Improves balance and coordination

- Makes labor pain, menstruation and menopause shorter and easier

- Massages internal organs

- Improves libido

Mental Benefits

- Save mind and body from devastating effects of daily stressors

- Yoga aids in development of coping skills

- Brings a positive outlook on life

- Yoga helps in overall development of soft skills

- Yoga helps with better mental well-being and clarity

- Calming of mind

- Better awareness

- Reduction of mild to severe stress patterns

- Sharpening of concentration

- Develops overall personality

- Increases will power and mental fortitude

- Aids learning efficiency

- Establishes self-discipline

- Treats mild to severe obsessive-compulsive disorders

Spiritual Benefits

- Brings in a sense of fulfillment

- Activates the body's energy centers

- Improves self-knowledge

- Manifests spiritual positivity

- Defines meaning and purpose of life

- Evokes inner consciousness

- Connects inner self to outer world

- Fosters sense of gratitude and appreciation

For you to derive these and many other benefits, you have to practice different yoga poses. In the subsequent chapters, we will discuss how to use yoga poses to achieve different goals.

Beginners Yoga Poses To Stretch And Bring In Flexibility

Since you are a complete beginner, it is perhaps important that we start by discussing beginner yoga poses in order to ease the learning process for you. Why is that important? Well, yoga is a discipline that requires your body to be lithe and bendable. Therefore, to start us off, we will discuss the poses that will help enhance your flexibility. Once these basic poses are mastered, we can graduate to higher and complex poses that will enable you to derive many more benefits while enhancing your experience as a yogi/yogini.

For starters, get a Yoga mat ready and wear comfortable attire. Lose clothes will not hinder the movements of your limbs while performing Yoga. In addition, do not eat at least half an hour before and after performing any of the yoga postures that we will be discussing in this book.

1. Mountain Pose

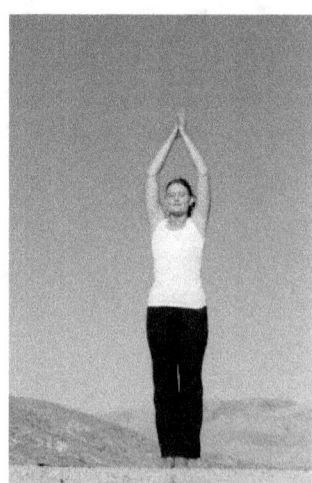

The Sanskrit name of this yoga pose is TADASANA. This posture is known to improve your body's posture, bring in mental clarity and regulate breathing pattern.

How to perform: Stand straight with your feet firmly placed on the ground and placed hip-wide apart. Allow the arms to rest on the sideways. Take slow and deep breaths while your neck is aligned at normal posture. Then slowly move both arms upward simultaneously and then join both palms over the head, akin to a mountain peak.

2. Warrior Pose

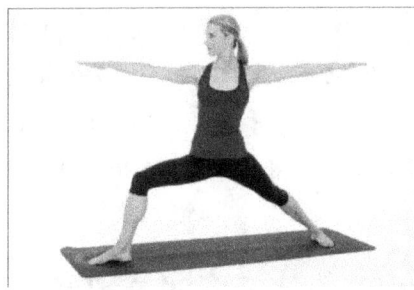

The Sanskrit name for this particular pose is VIRABHADRASANA. This yoga pose stretches and strengthens your limbs.

How to perform: Stand with a small gap between your feet. Then turn right while your right foot is at the angle of 90 degrees. Place your left foot slightly inward. As you do this, ensure to keep your shoulders stable. Extend both arms sideways while your arms are facing downwards. Slightly bend your right knee an angle of 90 degrees. Focus right on top of your arms for as long as possible. Repeat by switching sides.

3. Triangle Pose

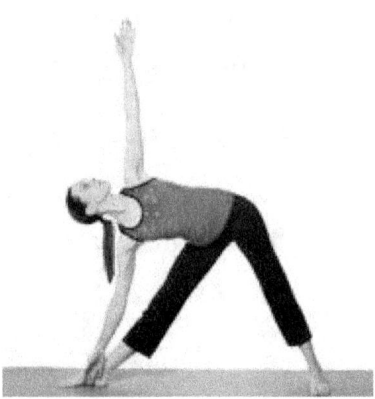

The Sanskrit name of this pose is TRIKONASAN. This pose helps a great deal in bringing flexibility to your body. It also strengthens joints and manages backache. Pregnant women are often advised to perform this pose to bring flexibility to their bodies.

How to perform: Perform the warrior pose when facing towards the left hand side without bending your knees. Now bend to the right and try to touch your right foot with the tips of your right hand fingertips. While doing this, your left hand should be reaching upwards. Switch sides.

Now that you've learnt how to perform basic yoga poses that enhance your flexibility, let's move on to the next bit, which is using yoga poses for other purposes like calming the mind.

Yoga Poses to Calm Your Mind

Our lives are full of stress and anxiety that tends to keep our mind ticking all the time. Consequently, an overworking mind tires itself and gets over-exhausted by thinking too much. As a well known saying goes – "It is all in mind"; our lives are largely controlled by our minds. Our minds hold immense power that drives our bodies all day long. In fact, it is rightly said that mental power can make a difference to our physical capacities.

Here is one example to prove that we can control our physical responses through our minds:

Close your eyes and imagine holding a shiny and a juicy lemon in your hand. You can feel the texture of the tangy fruit and how it is full of citrus juice. Now imagine slicing that lemon with a knife slowly and slowly. Imagine the sharp knife going inside the lemon and slitting it into two parts. Now imagine tasting the tangy lemon juice with your tongue.

Now open your eyes.

Didn't you start salivating as you imagined the above situation? I am sure you must have. Well, this is the power of our mind that is closely linked to our physical sensations and even pain control. When in pain, close your eyes and perceive your pain to be a lit candle. Now blow hard in imagination to put off the candle or watch it receding in the background. Soon, you will start feeling the lessening of pain.

Our mind and body work in tandem. While sleep relaxes our body, our mind often overworks and refuses to calm down amidst the hustle bustle of our busy lives. Gone are the days of uncomplicated and serene life when everything used to be simplified.

A layman has focus over the physical aspect of yoga, i.e. the poses. While Yoga poses do tone up and stretch our bodies, one unique yoga technique called 'drishti' (focusing the gaze) helps in calming the mind. When a yoga practitioner lays focus on a single point, his mind ceases to wander, as it would have no visual stimuli provided to it that would generate fidgety thoughts. In the absence of visual stimuli, the mind stays pure and less distracted.

The nervous system & yoga

Our bodies have two kinds of nervous systems. One is called - sympathetic system and the other is called parasympathetic system. Sympathetic nervous system (also known as "fight or flight" system) makes the blood pressure rise, increase the rate of breathing and generate stress related hormones. The stimulation of this system causes health issues like heart ailments, migraines, ulcers etc.

The second kind of nervous system is called parasympathetic. This nervous system is responsible for lowering down the blood pressure and for regulating the breathing pace. When blood pressure is controlled, it freely gets transmitted to the body's internal organs and systems, thus healing the damages and clearing the harmful build-ups.

Bringing in pranayam into the equation

Experts have proven that yoga poses and pranayam techniques encourage deep breathing that encourages the parasympathetic nervous system. This consequently leads to our mind's relaxation. If we compare a gym workout with a yoga session, we can clearly see that while in both the cases, the strength and flexibility is being gained; the yoga practitioner is reaping extra benefits of strengthening his/her 'parasympathetic' system. Working out in gym is just toning the body but practicing yoga is toning the body and calming the restless mind as well. Pranayam brings our attention towards breathing and makes us ponder over present happenings. We develop mindfulness and stay connected to now.

Yoga poses are best performed in tandem with the correct breathing pattern. The good news is that there are no short or quick breaths in yoga; rather, there are long and deep breaths. Relaxed and deep breathing while performing yoga poses changes our mental state making it calm and quiet. Thus, the combination of yoga poses, pranayama and and drishti (focusing) brings optimum physical health along with mental and emotional awareness.

Here are some poses that will greatly help you calm down your mind and harness its hidden potential. The suggested yoga poses will help you to find solace amidst the mental clutter, thus striking a balance between the mind and the body.

1. Eagle Pose

The Sanskrit name for this pose is Garundasana

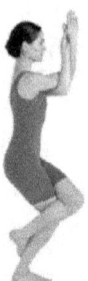

How to Perform: Find a spot in front of you and focus at that spot without moving. Take a deep breath and stay aware of your breathing pattern. Maintain the balance of your body. Now shift your body weight over the right foot. Cross over the right leg towards the left side for once or at most twice. Push your hips downward. Cover your right elbow with the left one along with the forearms. Press both palms firmly into one another. As your elbows are pressed in forward direction, stretch your fingers upwards. Take 5 deep breaths and repeat.

2. Dancer's Pose

The Sanskrit name for this pose is Natarajasana

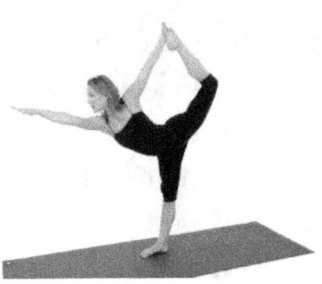

<u>How to Perform:</u> Stand firm on the ground with your feet slightly apart. Be mindful of your long and deep breaths. Lift one leg and stretch it backward, grabbing its toe-end with hand with the palm facing outward. Stretch the opposite arm in the front (as shown above) and then tilt your body to maintain balance. Allow your spine to get a soft curve by holding your feet in your palm. Take 4 to 5 deep breaths and shift sides.

<u>3. Child Pose</u>

The Sanskrit name for this pose is Balasana

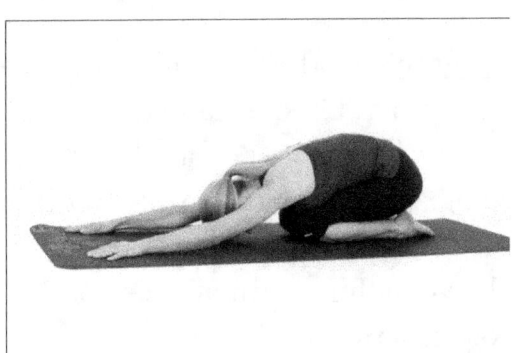

<u>How to Perform:</u> This relaxing pose can rejuvenate your physical and mental energy. Sit on a flat surface and kneel forward. Take a long and deep breath and then focus on

your breathing pattern. Do this while your knees are held together and your buttocks are resting on your feet. Lower down your torso towards your thighs then throw your breath outward and rest your hands on the surface. Stay in this position for 20 seconds. Gradually come back to the original position with regular breathing. Repeat 2 more times.

4. Forward Bend Pose

The Sanskrit name for this pose is Uttanasana

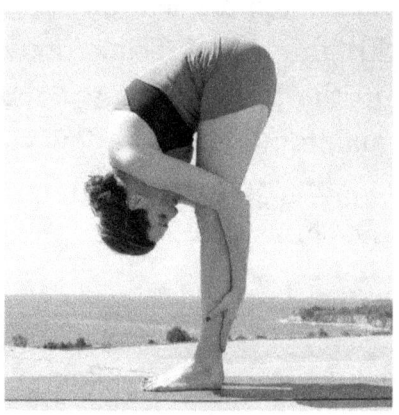

How to Perform: Stand erect while your feet are placed close to one another. Lift one hand upward and take a deep breath in. Now bend forward as you stretch your torso while exhaling. Use both hands to touch the ground as you keep your legs and knees straight. Stay in this pose for 20 seconds while breathing normally. Get back to the original position. Repeat 5 times.

5. Bridge Pose

The Sanskrit name for this pose is Setu Bandha Sarvangasana

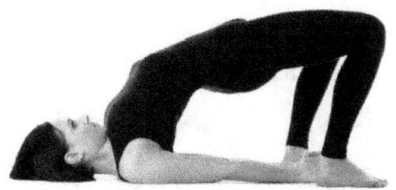

<u>How to Perform:</u> Lie on your back on a flat surface. Bend your knees and then place your feet in a resting position right next to your buttocks. As you do that, ensure to maintain relaxed and long breaths. Give support to your spine and lift your hips upwards. While rising upward, lift up your breastbone and press your arms to the floor. Let your eyes be fixed to the ceiling. Stay in this pose for 20 seconds and then gradually come back to the original position. Repeat 5 times.

<u>6. Cat Pose</u>

The Sanskrit name for this pose is Marjaryasana

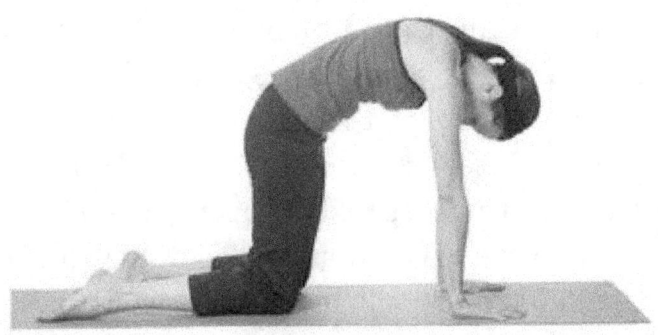

Get on your four limbs then take a deep breath and exhale after a while. Your wrists should be placed directly under your shoulders and while your knees should be placed right under your hips. Exhale and then curve your spine inward. This will in turn point your spine outward towards the ceiling. Now bend your head and bring your chin close to the breast. However, your chin should not be touching the breast. Stay in this pose for 20 seconds and slowly come back to the original position. Repeat the pose 5 times. During the pose, stay focused towards your breathing pattern.

7. Corpse Pose

The Sanskrit name for this pose is Savasana

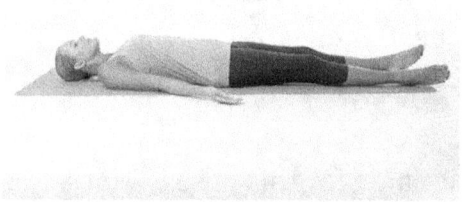

This is the ultimate yoga pose for soothing the mind. Lie down on a firm and a comfortable surface. If needed, place a soft pillow or a cushion to support your head. Allow your feet to stay slightly apart from one another while keeping your toes and knees relaxed. Your arms should be placed sideways and palms should be open and facing upward. Now close your eyes gently and take soft breaths. Feel your breath and relax your mind and body. You can be in this pose for 10 to 12 minutes. Ideally, this should be the last pose of your yoga session.

Dissolve Stress with Yoga Nidra

Stress is the monster we all live with. It has invaded our personal and professional lives and refuses to budge from there. Nonetheless, the truth is that our daily stressors determine the quality of lives we lead. In particular, they strip us of our daily joys that we miss in the quest of unseen happiness. We wait for future events that would give us happiness in futility and omit the present times that hold the secret of our happiness and contentment. Neither can we reverse our unpleasant past events that have been the prime cause of stress nor can we predict our future that causes us anxiety. We can choose to be happy by dissolving our stress. Here is how to go about it:

Yoga nidra

Yoga nidra is the deep relaxation yoga technique that gives your mind and body a wonderful rejuvenation. It works at healing our body and mind of its daily stressors and their side effects. For instance, problems like hypertension and insomnia are due to the stress build-up in our mind. This yoga technique, when practiced, brings down the level of tension and makes us more productive. But how does this yoga technique enable us to achieve all that?

Science Behind Yoga nidra

Yoga nidra is a wonderful amalgamation of profound relaxation and mindful awareness. It allows effortless tapping of our mind's inherent creativity, intuition and abundance. Yoga nidra is backed by science facts for silencing the mental clattering. For instance, it absorbs usual consciousness, drops down your brain's rhythm and submerges into alpha state. Here are some more facts –

- Yoga nidra brings focus of all energies towards the inner sanctuary (third eye) that is located between the eyebrows. This brings down the level of stress.

- Yoga nidra accesses the insightfulness of right side of your brain along with logic of left side of the brain. This integrates relaxation with simultaneous mindfulness.

- The focus over the third eye activates the center part of your brain and stimulates the pineal gland. This gland releases a hormone named melatonin that prevents sickness, reduces anxiety, keeps nervous system healthy and brings in restful sleep.

- Medical experts have used EEG (Electroencephalograph) to conclude that post Yoga nidra, there is increase of alpha brain waves that relaxes your body's nervous system.

- Regular practicing of Yoga nidra reduces stress hormones and brings down heart rate & blood pressure

- Yoga Nidra ushers the practitioner into a subconscious sleep state where there is relaxed brainwave activity. This is the state where a conscious intersection can be made from left brain's logic to right brain's intuitiveness.

Yoga nidra aims at guided relaxation that takes a practitioner into a deep state of rest. The body gets relaxed while the mind visualizes soothing imagery. Here is a step-by-step guide on how to practice yoga nidra.

- ✓ After you have performed your yoga session successfully, cover your body with a thin blanket to retain the body's heat. A sudden drop in your body's temperature at the time of performing yoga nidra will not be suitable.

- ✓ Select a peaceful and a quiet room for an undisturbed session of yoga nidra session. Lie down on your back in the corpse Pose (Shavasana) and close your eyes gently. Relax your mind and maintain a slow and steady breathing pattern. In case you feel pain in back, you can use a thin pillow or cushion to support you.

- ✓ Bring your attention and focus over your right foot for a couple of seconds. Gradually, move your attention upward to the right calf, right knee, right thigh and right hip. Awaken your awareness towards the right side of your body.

- ✓ Repeat above procedure for your left side body parts.

- ✓ Now move your attention to the remaining body parts like the stomach, genital parts, navel, chest, right shoulder and right arm. Follow same procedure for your left shoulder, left arm, face, throat and finally the crown of your head.

✓ Take a deep breath in and observe what happens to your bodily sensations. Stay relaxed in this tranquil state for the next few minutes.

✓ Gradually, awaken your awareness towards your surroundings. Gently turn towards your right side and lie for some more seconds.

✓ Slowly get up, sit, and open your eyes when you feel like.

As you practice yoga, you will realize that you may need to learn a few practices that will enhance your ability to derive the most yoga benefits. One such practice is chanting the AUM mantra. Let's discuss what this is all about in the next chapter.

AUM Chanting: Awakening of The Mind and Body

AUM Chant

AUM is a powerful syllable that holds immense creative power and spiritual significance. Also chanted as 'Om', AUM is the sound of entirety that vibrates in the universe and brings in calmness and peace to the body and mind.

When we chant the syllable AUM, our bodily and spiritual intuitiveness gets awakened. It merges the vibrations of the universe and the body to surcharge our comprehensive existence with divinity.

The syllable AUM represents the supreme power of our Creator. Try chanting any name – of a person, a thing or an animal – you won't find any inspiration seeping in. Now try chanting AUM in continuity and feel the development of divine perception within your mind and soul. Your vision gets enlarged and your mental horizon gets broadened.

How to Chant AUM

✓ The very first step towards chanting AUM is to find a calm and a secluded place where there would be no disturbance. Sit comfortably on a firm surface, preferably on the ground. Sit cross-legged and keep your spine straight.

✓ Ensure that you are wearing comfortable clothing in order to stay relaxed and focused.

✓ Cup your palms in your lap. Your left palm should hold the right palm, keeping it facing upward.

✓ Close your eyes gently and take deep breaths. Keep your body and mind relaxed and free of distractions.

✓ Take note of your subtle bodily vibrations.

✓ Now take a long breath in within the count of 5 seconds. Hold your breath for 5 seconds and then exhale. Take 7 seconds to exhale.

✓ Repeat this breathing pattern for 3 times.

✓ At the time of exhalation for the 3rd time, produce sounds by vibrating your epiglottal zone. You should feel the vibrations under your chest area.

✓ On full exhalation, relax for a few seconds.

✓ Again, inhale and start chanting "Aaaaauuuuummm..." Spend nearly 80 percent of the exhalation span in chanting "Aaaauuuu" and the remaining 20 percent should be for chanting just "mmmmmmm".

✓ Repeat the above steps 3 times and gradually increase.

✓ Now relax and focus on normal pace of your breathing for 3 to 4 minutes.

Tips & Suggestions for AUM Chanting

- Do not sit in strong sunlight or windy surroundings. You want your body and mind to be free from any form of distractions.

- Do not consume alcohol for at least 7 to 8 hours before starting.

- Do not eat a heavy meal 2 hours before the chanting so that your digestive channel does not get blocked.

- As a beginner, you may feel dizzy or nauseated. To avoid that, go slow in such cases and allow time for your mind and body to get accustomed.

- Keep your eyes gently closed and open after you have regained your normal breath.

Benefits of AUM Chanting

AUM chanting brings about many benefits. Let us discuss those with a scientific explanation:

- Dispels depression and anxiety

- Unblocks mind-body circuits and restores energy flow

- AUM chanting can help you balance your hormones, which subsequently help you to fight stress, anxiety and depression.

- AUM chanting brings in console and relieve

- AUM chanting liberates us from earthly and unfulfilled desires

- It soothes on a cellular level with devotional surrender

- Turns negative perception into positive

- Frees restless minds from self-inflicted grief

- Awakens our heart and evokes compassion to set free off envy, animosity, and pride

- Boosts immunity by regulating communication between the body's endocrine system and the nervous system

- Helps in adjusting bodily rhythms that keep on happening inside our bodies round the clock and tend to go offbeat due to daily stressors

- Opens creativity and intuition due to the activation of hypothalamus signals

In nutshell, AUM chanting dissolves our egos into unison, the very essence of yoga. Our thoughts become refined that further elevate our perceptions for a brilliant inner and outer radiance.

Scientific Backing of AUM Chant

It is important to state here that AUM is believed to be a universal syllable that doesn't refer to any particular God or divinity sect. Indeed, it is a traditional concept but it is backed by science.

- The AUM chanting causes vibrations that result in unique effects with each syllable –

    o Chanting of "aaaaaaaaaa" resonates with the nervous system zone that affects our chest and stomach region.

    o Chanting of "oooooooooo" causes sensations in the chest and throat region

    o Chanting of "mnnnmmm" activates the brain region and the nasal cavity

- The concatenation of AUM in a sequentially pattern activates our internal organs like spinal cord, stomach, throat, brain and nasal region. The energy moves upward from the abdominal area and activates our spinal cord.

- The results of time-frequency analysis revealed that prior to regular chanting of AUM syllable, the brain's cardiogram pattern was abrupt and wavy. The same experiment was repeated after regular chanting of AUM and the results showed drastic improvement where the waveforms became regularly spaced and symmetrical. The participants found their state of mind to be calm and peaceful.

- Scientists have successfully analyzed MRI results before and after AUM chanting. Regular chanting of

AUM syllable has effectively treated epilepsy, low blood pressure and even severe depression.

Hence, AUM chanting has scientific backing that is known to bring benefits in the form of mental agility, curing of stress & depression, improvement in concentration and overall happiness.

Conclusion

Thank you again for purchasing this book!

I hope this book was able to help you to understand how to use yoga to fight stress, anxiety and be happy.

Now is the time to put what you have learnt into practice.

Thank you and good luck!